MAKING FACES

DENNIE PASION

PHOTOGRAPHS BY URSULA STEIGER

QUADRILLE

contents

INTRODUCTION **3**

ABOUT THE BASICS **6**

FINGERPAINTING **12**

MAKE YOURSELF UP . . . **14**
[24 STUNNING LOOKS TO FIRE THE IMAGINATION]

USEFUL ITEMS **62**

WHERE TO BUY **63**

ACKNOWLEDGEMENTS **64**

introduction

Real Beauty is understanding the many facets of who you are and being true to your own developing beliefs, dreams, and character. Make-up has been referred to as a mask, a ritual, or a subtle enhancement of natural beauty. I prefer to think of my make-up as the spark of energy igniting a state of being.

Who you are and how you present yourself today may not be the same tomorrow: a change of face reflects the way you feel or how you want to be seen. MAKING FACES presents compositions in colour, texture and design, to encourage you to explore not only what suits you, but to experiment with who you wish to be. There are no complicated brush strokes, just simple suggestions to fire the imagination. Design a look and then seal it with your own fingerprints.

The looks have been inspired by people from many cultures whom I have been fortunate to meet, including the Aborigines of Australia, the Samburu of Kenya, and the Zulu of South Africa, and I would like to pay tribute to their philosophy and spirit. I associate colours mainly with experiences I have had in countries the world over: to me, Egypt is green, India is pink, Mexico is blue; but the most beautiful rainbow I have ever seen was in East Acton, London. Wherever you are, be Inspired.

Experiment with the unexpected and follow no rules. Have no fear, have fun, be yourself . . .

Dennie Pasion

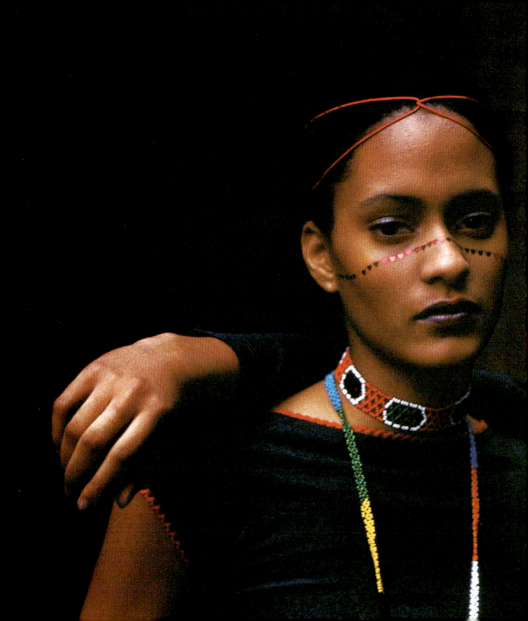

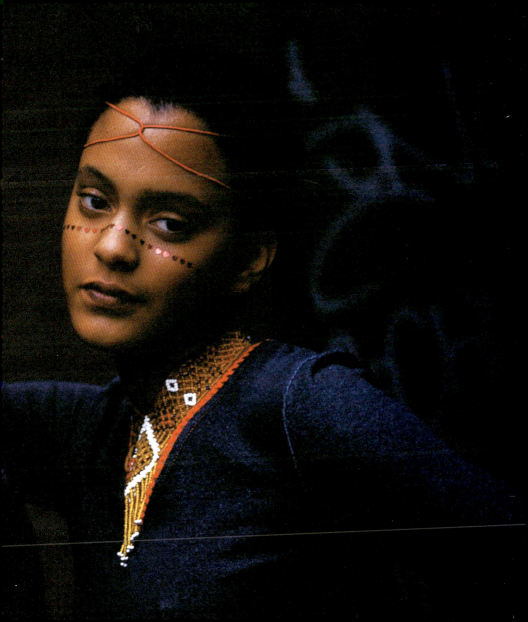

about the basics...

laying the foundation

basic foundation types:
3-in-1 foundation / concealer / powder – for maximum coverage
Duo compact – use wet or dry
Liquid – for a sheer finish
Tinted moisturizer – light and transparent

HOT TIP: ALWAYS MOISTURIZE AFTER CLEANSING AND BEFORE FOUNDATION FOR A SMOOTH AND EVEN FINISH.

Foundation creates a blank canvas for design. The perfect foundation feels light to the touch, and covers, but still reveals the skin's natural complexion. It takes time to choose a foundation but fortunately there are many good products available in all price ranges that not only cover extremely well but also moisturize and protect. It is not necessary to use a foundation if your skin is healthy and you want to create a natural look. Fresh skin, moisturized and glowing, looks amazing without a base, as in Barefaced. If your skin is a little patchy and you experience breakout, consider covering only these areas by dabbing lightly with foundation or concealer.

SELECTION: Make sure your foundation is easy to use: jars can be awkward and messy, and product can be wasted – once you have dipped in your fingers, it is contaminated and will not last. It will also need to be portable if you want to be able to take it with you on nights out.

One of the most important things to ensure is that your foundation matches your skin's natural pigment: avoid orange or pink tones in a foundation as they are difficult to blend. For a fresh pink flush or a sunkissed glow, use blush or bronzing powder over a natural base. During the summer, you may wish to use a tinted moisturizer with sunscreen rather than a heavy foundation, particularly if you like to look slightly tanned.

Foundation coats the skin and so it is important that the foundation you choose allows your skin to breathe, except for those one-off theatrical looks, such as Lovebite or Wicked, where it is more effective to create a mask-like appearance.

HOT TIP: USE A WATER-SOLUBLE CLEANSER WHICH CAN BE RINSED OFF WITH TEPID WATER.

APPLICATION: Moisturize skin; blot excess with a tissue. Using a damp sponge, or your two middle fingers, apply foundation, beginning on forehead. Work from the centre out using the quick blending motion of press, twist and release (see page 12). [If you use sweeping movements the foundation will end up collecting around the edge of the face.] It does take practise so check your blending around jawbone and hair line. Coat a puff with translucent powder and press and pat over the face to set make-up for a matte finish.

concealing the truth

Sometimes concealers are necessary to minimize dark shadows under eyes or to cover blemishes. It is possible to find a foundation that also acts as a concealer, although concealer should normally be one shade lighter than your base or natural skin tone.

APPLICATION: For under the eye: dab a little onto the back of your hand, wait a few seconds as if it is setting, and then, with your little finger, gently press along the shadowed areas under the eyes. For blemishes: using the tip of a small brush, dab the blemish avoiding the skin around it. Then dab onto the spot once, with your little finger, and the concealer should blend whilst keeping the blemish covered.

lip service

basic lipstick types:
Matte – strong, textured, intense colour with no shine
Creme – softer colours with texture and little shine
Gloss – use alone for illuminated shine or over matte lipstick
Transparent – a stain with no texture

HOT TIP: FOR A FRESH NATURAL LOOK, OUTLINE THE LIP WITH A NEUTRAL PENCIL, POUT AS IF BLOWING A KISS, THEN PRESS A GLOSS OR TRANSPARENT INTO THE POUT WITH THE INDEX FINGER.

Lips are the frame of your voice and should always look soft and smooth. Eyes and lips are the beacons of inner health and lips should be cleansed and moisturized along with the skin.

PROTECTING: Lips that are in great shape are much easier to paint. If your lips are dry or flaky, gently exfoliate with a soft toothbrush to remove roughness and dead skin. Drink lots of water and try not to use lip balms as they can dry out the lips. Vitamin E in balm lipstick or creme is excellent for healthy lips. Elizabeth Arden's eight hour creme (see page 63) is a great investment as a moisturizer – it is also very good for bites, dry skin, sunburn and nail cuticles. Trūcco's Lip Perfect is also a good primer, softening lips before lipstick is applied.

APPLICATION: For a fuller, larger lip, use a neutral lip pencil to draw a line on the outer edge of the lip line, then fill in with lipstick up to the pencil line. Take care not to go over the line as this will look unnatural. Lips that have been primed with a vitamin E creme may just need a little lipstick blended with the index finger or smudged across the centre of the lip. Along with the four basic lipstick types shown above, there are also 3-in-1 cremes that can be used all over the face, including over the lips. If you choose to use a transparent, you will need to test first as they often look lighter on the lip than the packaging suggests. If you are creating more dramatic, matte lips, always use a brush with a steady hand and blot with a tissue before reapplying. Matte lips can be set with a little translucent powder.

Dabbing a little gloss in the centre of dramatic lips creates subtle shine, without causing the lip colour to bleed or smudge. When blotting, bite into a tissue with the lips to avoid getting lipstick on your teeth. If you wish to shape the lips, shade the corners darker with a pencil or matte lipstick and then use a lighter, glossier shade for the centre. Most of the lipsticks used in MAKING FACES are gloss and transparents as these are easier to apply using the fingers.

the cheek of it

basic blush types:
Creme – intense colour, good for layering and for dry skin
Gel – transparent, for shine
Powder – matte, for shape and control

HOT TIP: SHINY CHEEKBONES CREATE A LOOK OF VITALITY, AS IN RUSH: SHINE IN THE CENTRE OF THE CHEEK GIVES THE ILLUSION OF ROUND, HOT CHEEKS

Subtle blush can change a mood and transform a look. If your skin is in good condition, it is fun to layer with the different textures of creme, gel and powder. You can apply blush over fresh, dewy, moisturized skin, although it can blend more easily over foundation. Concentrate product on areas where you would blush naturally.

APPLICATION: To apply powder blush, press in and smooth out. To apply gels, press and pat, working in circular motions around the cheek and up towards the temples. To apply cremes, lightly smooth colour over the cheeks, layering for more intensity of colour. For contouring and highlighting, suck in the cheeks and apply product using the outer cushion of the palm of your hand, or a large brush, working from the upper part of the hollow out. For an all over sunkissed glow, brush colour in a circular motion clockwise over face, throat, and forehead, as in Heatwave. The simple way to apply perfect blush is to smile and then apply blush to the apple of the cheek.

the eye of the storm

basic eye shadow types:
Creme – multi-purpose, for smudging and blending
Stick – easy to apply, for highlighting and contouring
Powdered colouration – for more control and intensity of colour

HOT TIP: TAKE A COUPLE OF COTTON BUDS WITH YOU WHEN YOU'RE OUT, TO CLEAN INNER CORNERS OF THE EYE THAT COLLECT EYELINER AND POWDER.

HOT TIP: WHEN USING BLACK EYE SHADOW OR DARK SHADES, PRESS LOOSE POWDER UNDER EYE AREA TO CATCH PARTICLES THAT COULD POSSIBLY FALL AND SMEAR. WHEN EYE MAKE-UP IS FINISHED, DUST POWDER AWAY GENTLY WITH A SOFT BRUSH.

Eyes are the windows to the soul; with make-up you can send out signals of what lies within. You can easily create a trademark look that enhances your individual eye colour or shape: mascara and extra lashes; a beauty spot two inches below the outer corner of your left eye; or an Egyptian influence in your eyeliner shape. Looks that work well are examples of contradiction and juxtaposition: bright citrus eyes with dramatic dark lips; smouldering metallic eyes constrasting with clear lip gloss.

APPLICATION: For a clear, open eye, dab white eye shadow into the corners of the eyes and line inner rim with white pencil. For a sharper outline and slimmer shape, line inner rim with black pencil and smudge under the outer corners with brown or black shadow. If eyeliner looks too harsh, soften with dark brown shadow brushed over the line, or smudge with a knuckle. To contour eyes, shade with darker tones under brow bone into the eye socket; to highlight, use pale shades above brow bone in corners and centre of lid.

MASCARA

Always use an eye make-up remover to dissolve mascara before cleansing. Do not keep mascara for too long as it can become thick and flaky; two months is about the limit. If you want to use an eyelash curler, it is better to use plastic rather than metal, which can be too harsh, and always use the curler before you have applied mascara. Transparent colourless mascara is wonderful for healthy long lashes, and there is a large variety of mascara

HOT TIP: USE CONCEALER ON THE EYELID TO SEE TRUE TONES AND COLOURS IN EYE SHADOW.

HOT TIP: TRY EYE SHADOW ON THE BROW FOR A SOFTER EFFECT, AND USE DIFFERENT COLOURS TO CREATE DRAMA.

colours now available, so you can experiment and create an individual look. After applying mascara, comb the lashes through with an eyelash comb to separate the lashes and eliminate blobs.

EYEBROWS

If you feel you need to reshape your brows, only pluck from under the brow, never above. Natural eyebrows look great almost always, but if the brow creates too much shadow over the eye it can make you look tired. Most of the time you may only need to clear away a few fine hairs that can make your eye shadow clog up slightly under your brow. Shapes change with the seasons so if you want a lot of shaping, seek the advice and expertise of a professional. Create new looks with colour, pencils and accessories, as in Flybrow. To use a pencil, brush brows first to shape them and then fill in with a pencil, blending with a knuckle.

about the looks...

The symbols shown for each look give information on application technique (see pages 12-13) and the colour of the product used. If you cannot, or do not wish to find the specified product through the information on pages 62-64, these symbols will help you match the colour with an alternative product, either from your own make-up bag or from a different make-up range. Let the combination of colours and techniques used for these looks inspire your own special creations.

fingerpainting

  use your **MIDDLE FINGER** (left) for smoothing foundation and blush. For more even coverage of product use the **MIDDLE AND RING FINGERS TOGETHER** (right) to press and smooth make-up, blending it into the skin using press, twist and release: press into the skin, twist the fingers quickly and lightly, and release.

 use your **RING FINGER** to achieve more intensity of colour. With the fingertip apply colour to the eyelids by pressing and patting rather than smoothing. Try layering different colours or textures for dramatic effects.

 use your **LITTLE FINGER** to pat and smooth make-up around the delicate eye areas, for instance pat concealer gently under the corner of the eye, down and away. Also use for blending and smudging colour under lower lashes.

 use the **PAD ON THE SIDE OF YOUR PALM** for contouring: either under the chin, around the temples or feel directly under the cheekbone and smooth colour upwards.

use a **BRUSH** (left) or **PENCIL** (right)
for shape, control, and density of colour,
or for more defined lines around the lips and eyes.

use your **INDEX FINGER** for smoothing lip gloss or
lipstick onto lips and for smoothing colour onto the eyelids.
Smoothing is a gentle application movement backwards
and forwards until the surface reflects an even blend of colour.

use your **KNUCKLE** to smear and smudge
colour under or over the outer corner of the eye.
Use with liquid eyeliner, eyeliner pencil, cremes or powders.

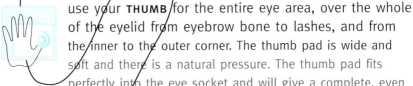

use your **THUMB** for the entire eye area, over the whole of the eyelid from eyebrow bone to lashes, and from the inner to the outer corner. The thumb pad is wide and soft and there is a natural pressure. The thumb pad fits perfectly into the eye socket and will give a complete, even coverage of colour with one or two sweeps.

Use the thumb technique by pressing the pad firmly into your colour (which might be a jumbo crayon, lipstick, creme shadow, concealer gel or eye powder colouration) and apply to the eye, starting at the inner corner and then sweeping out.

freckles&fatlashes

LIPS
Maybelline Icy Beige

FOUNDATION
Maybelline True Illusion

CHEEKS
Maybelline Raspberry Whisper

MASCARA
Maybelline Illegal Lengths

Draw lines under lashes with Rimmel Jet Black eye pencil. Draw white lines in between the black with Max Factor Wicked White pencil. Dot freckles over nose with Rimmel Brown eye pencil.

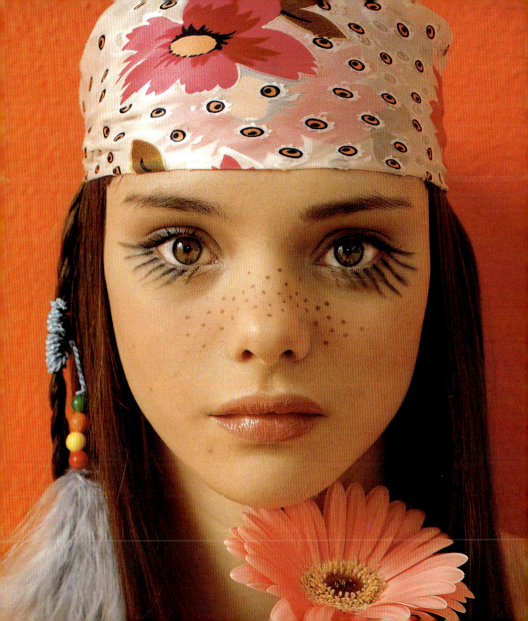

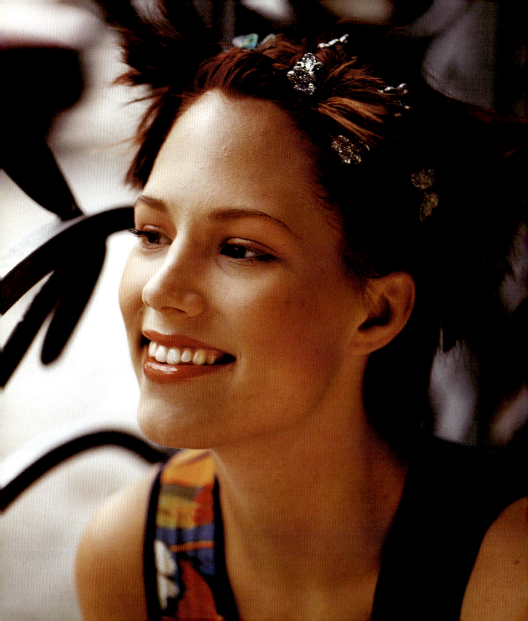

EYES Colourings
Golden Pearl and Sandstone

EYES Rimmel Special Eyes
Spirit and Brulee

LIPS Rimmel lasting finish Bare

FOUNDATION Max Factor 3-in-1
complete makeup Soft Beige

CHEEKS Rimmel Sun Shimmer
natural bronzer

MASCARA Rimmel endless lash Brown

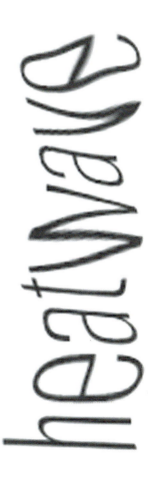

heatwave

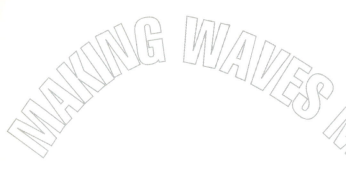

FOUNDATION Maybelline True Illusion

EYES L'Oréal Raging Violet

UNDEREYE L'Oréal Super Liner Purple

EYE WAVE L'Oréal Super Liner Purple

LIPS L'Oréal Rouge Pulp Violet Desire

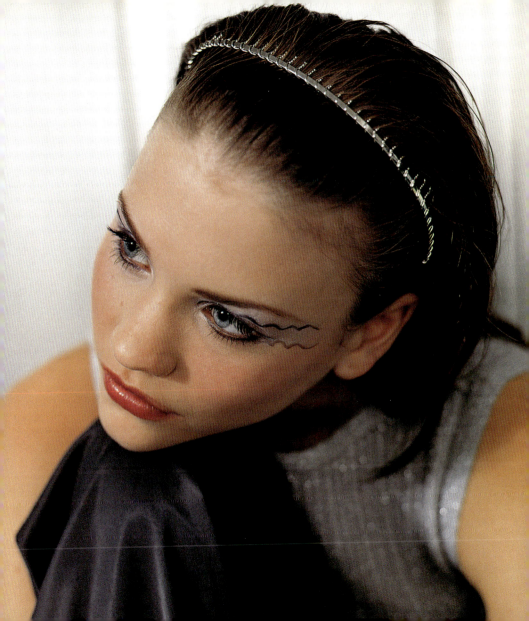

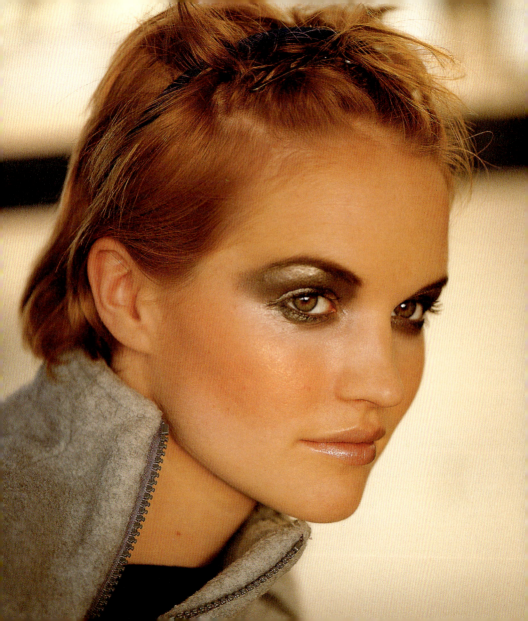

FOUNDATION Trūcco Bisque

CHEEKS Trūcco Flirt

EYES Trūcco Dark Angel Reflective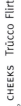

EYES Trūcco Venus Reflective

UNDER EYE Trūcco Dark Angel and Venus

LIPS Trūcco Ingenue

metal ice

EYES orange from Ben Nye wheel

LIPS orange from Ben Nye wheel, mixed with clear gloss

THE KIT: L'Oréal Identité Mehndi brush and black and white inks (see page 62) or Max Factor Jet Black and Wicked White eye pencils, bhindi or other stick-on accessory (see page 62).

Over the top of the orange colour on eyes and brow, paint (or draw) your design freehand using the Identité inks (or the Max Factor eye pencils): paint black lines first and then highlight with white. Once you are happy with the result, stick the bhindi, or chosen accessory, onto your forehead to complete the look.

free spirit ○ ● ●

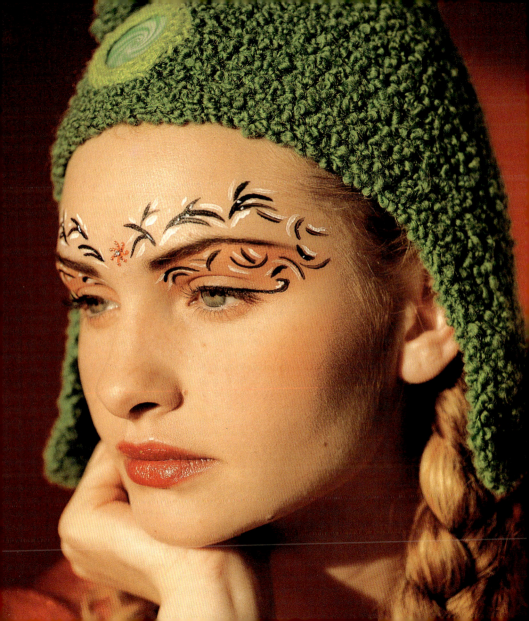

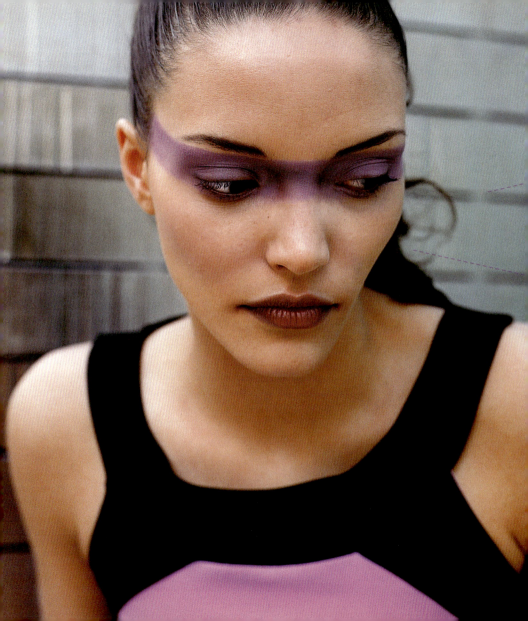

cosmic eye ray

EYE BAND Colourings Eye Shine Lavender (be generous with application)

LIPS Rimmel High Frost Storm

EYE BAND, SECOND COAT Trúcco Ecstasy Reflective

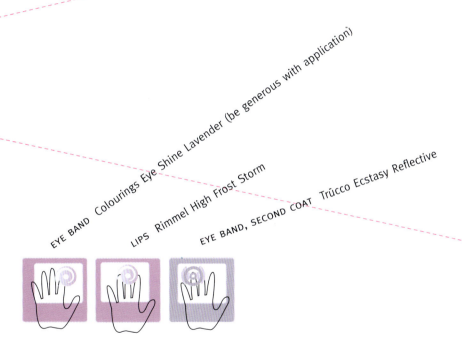

Using a ruler, draw a line with a neutral eye pencil directly across the eyelids and bridge of the nose, just below the brow. Placing the ruler parallel with the top of the ear, draw another line under the eye. Match and complete the lines so that the band is even from ear to ear. Fill in with colours as above.

summer breeze

FOUNDATION
Max Factor tinted moisturizer

CHEEKS
Maybelline Sierra Sand

EYES
Max Factor Passion

INNER CORNER OF EYES
Maybelline Cool Mint

OUTER CORNER OF EYES
Maybelline Cool Mint

LIPS Trucco Coy

MASCARA Maybelline Great Lash

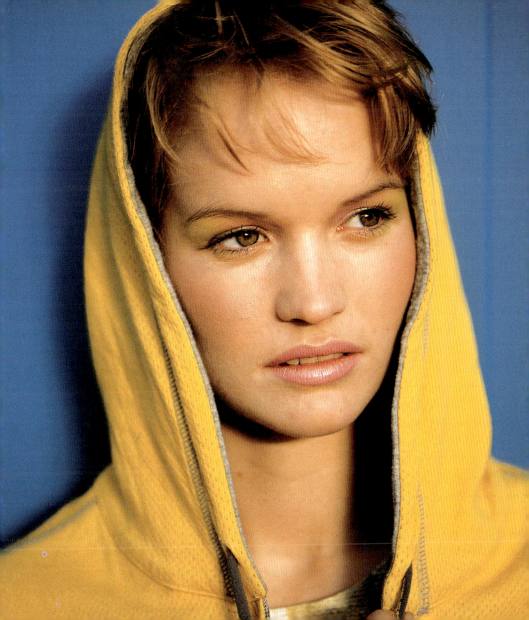

Lipstick Quick   EYES LIPS AND CHEEKS

THE KIT: neutral lip or eye pencil, lip brush, powder puff, translucent face powder, yellow crayon (or the yellow from the Ben Nye wheel), red lipstick in either Rimmel, High Frost Diva or Trūcco, Chilli Pepper (or the red from the Ben Nye wheel – see page 62).

Draw a flame shape on the eyelids with the pencil. Using a brush, fill in lips and flame with your chosen red. Dab the powder puff into the powder and pat over eyes and lips. Dust off the excess and re-apply the red. Draw yellow around the flame with a crayon, or paint on with a brush if using the Ben Nye wheel. Finally, smudge a little of the red over the apple of the cheek.

RAD

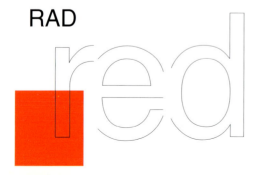

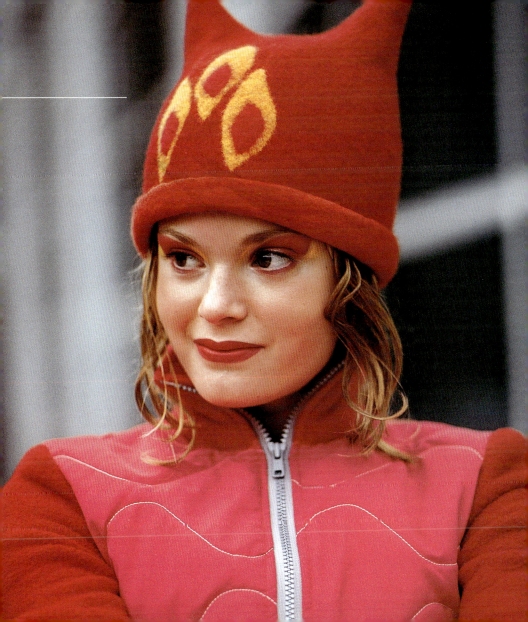

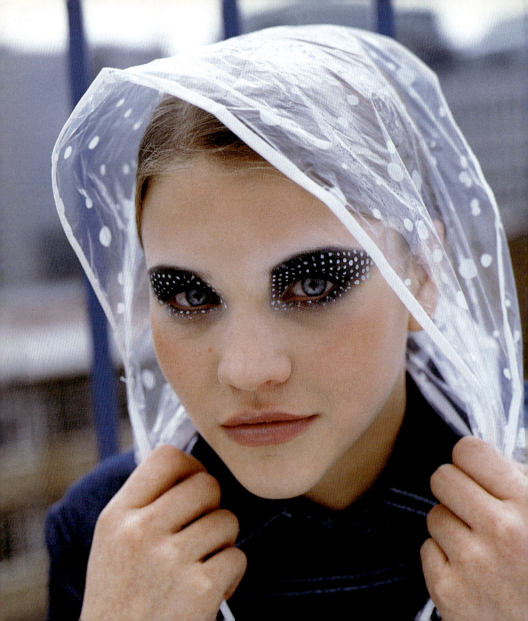

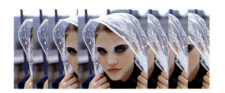

digital eye movement

Thumb L'Oréal Shantung Black eye shadow over eye area. Paint white dots freehand with L'Oréal Identité Mehndi brush and white ink (see page 62) or dot with Max Factor Wicked White pencil.

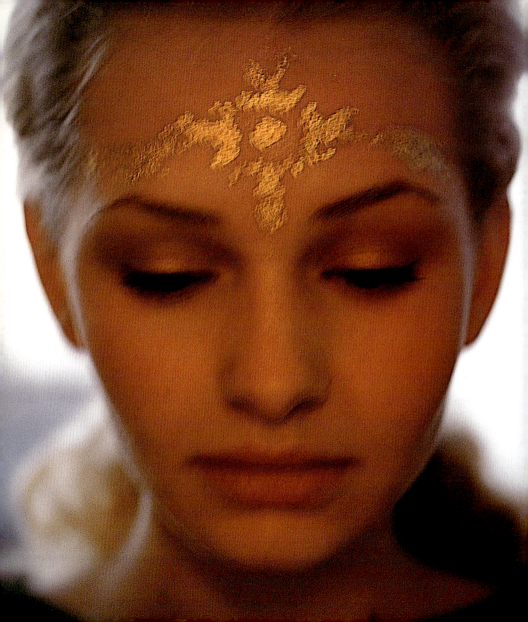

Celtic Gold

THE KIT: one sheet of gold leaf, vaseline or lip gloss.

CHOOSING YOUR PATTERN: either buy a stencil (see page 62) or make your own pattern from a celtic or other symbol, drawing the design onto paper and cutting it out to use as a template. You can also draw a freehand design directly onto your forehead.

Cover the area you want to decorate with a thick and sticky layer of vaseline or lip gloss. If using a stencil or template press it to the forehead, then press the gold leaf firmly over the sticky area. Pull the paper away very carefully, leaving the gold leaf stuck to the gloss in an amazing pattern. If using a freehand design, dab the gold leaf directly onto the sticky areas. To remove, just wipe off with a tissue.

WARNING — KEEP GOLD LEAF AWAY FROM THE EYES; DO NOT APPLY WITHOUT HAVING FIRST DONE A SKIN TEST

mesmerise

THE KIT: regular sized teaspoon, black eye pencil, translucent powder, bhindis or other accessories. TO DRAW THE EYE DESIGN: cup the eye with the spoon, draw a line with eye pencil around the top curve of the spoon and along the handle. Wipe the spoon before doing the other eye, and take care that the lines above the eyes are level. Use the spoon handle again to create a second straight line underneath the first. For more definition around the eyes, line the rims of your eyes with pencil. Dab with a little translucent powder to prevent smudging. Stick accessories on lines and forehead.

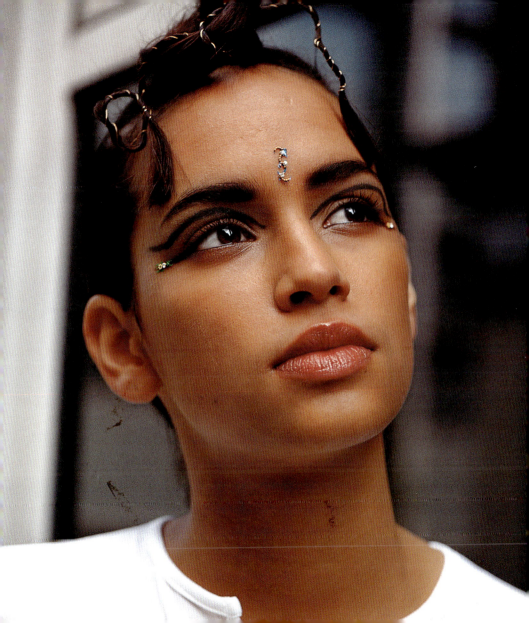

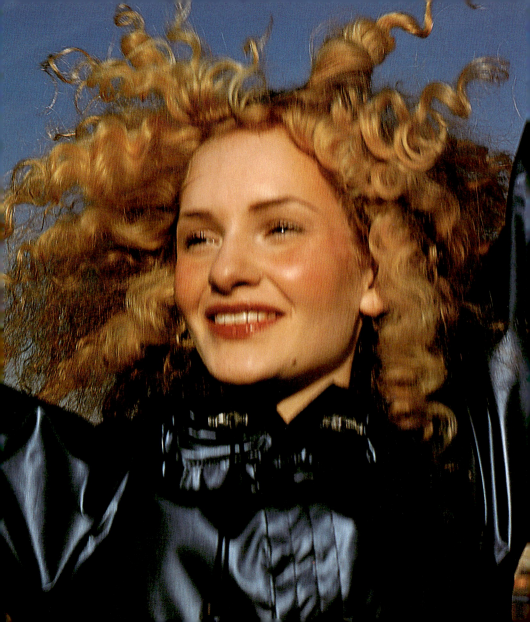

FOUNDATION
Trūcco tinted moisturizer

CHEEKS AND CHEEK BONES
mix and layer with Trūcco Transpigment

EYES
mix and layer with Trūcco Translating

LIPS
mix colours from above

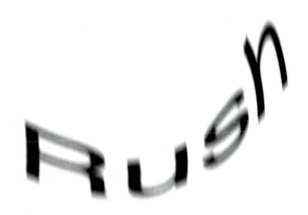

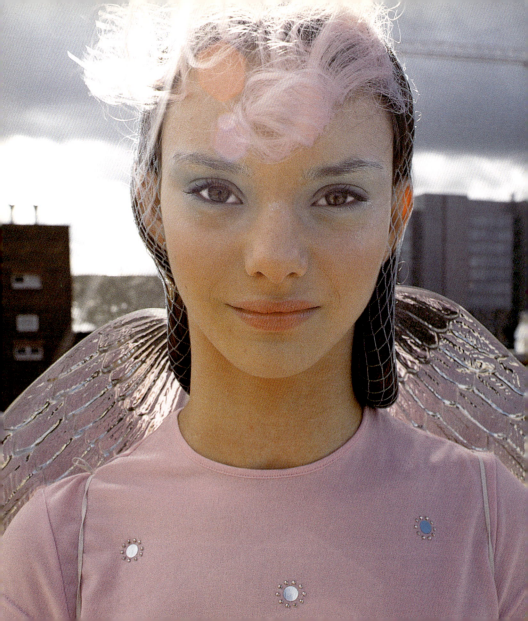

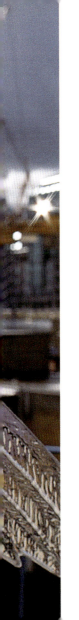

EYES
Rimmel Special Eyes Enterprise

EYES
Rimmel Special Eyes Enterprise

EYES
Rimmel Special Eyes Waterfall

FOUNDATION
Trūcco Porcelain Ivory

EYES AND CHEEKBONES
Max Factor shimmer stick

urban angel

Apply vaseline, lip gloss or eight hour creme (see page 8) to the eyelids before adding any glitter. Dab glitter onto the areas that you have primed, using blue, copper, green, red, gold, and silver glitter as desired (see page 62).

WARNING – KEEP GLITTER AWAY FROM LASHES AND DO NOT USE BODY GLITTER AROUND EYES

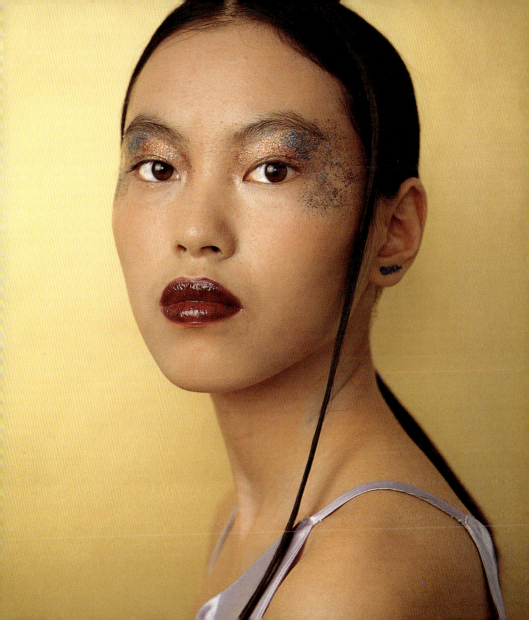

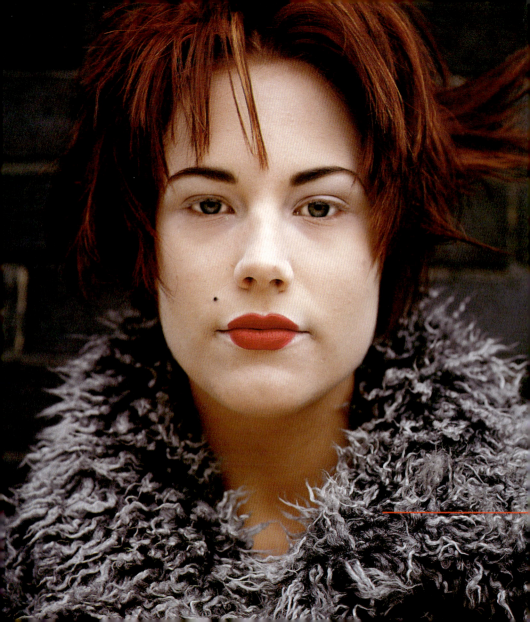

EYES Colourings highlighter stick Eclipse

 FOUNDATION Colourings All in One face base 01

 EYEBROWS AND BEAUTY SPOT Rimmel Jet Black pencil

 LIPS Apply Ben Nye Clown White (see page 62) over the corners of your mouth. Draw a cupid bow over your lips with red lip pencil. Paint in lips with Colourings Ruby Red.

LoVeBITe

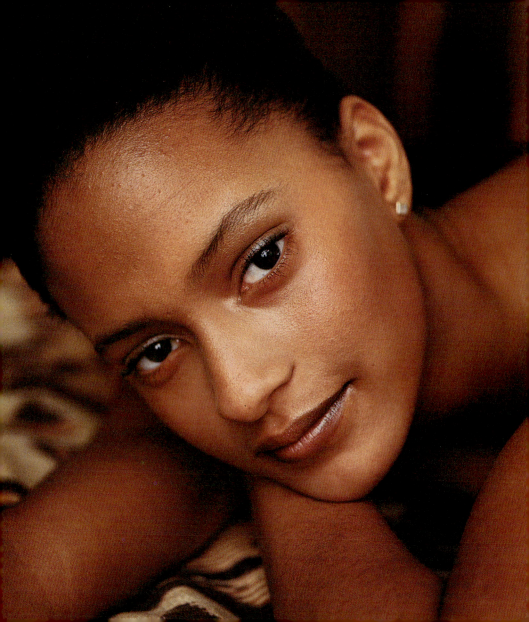

EYES Maybelline
Great Wear eyecolour 40

CHEEKS, BROW, JAWBONE AND EYES
Colourings Complete Colour Bronze

CHEEKS, BROW, JAWBONE AND EYES
Max Factor Moonbeam

LIPS Rimmel Birthday Suit

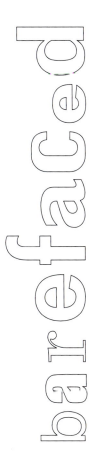

LIPS PAINTED Trûcco Wicked

INNER AND OUTER RIMS OF EYES Rimmel Jet Black pencil

UNDER EYE AND TO OUTLINE FLAME Max Factor Royal pencil
EYES, UNDER BROW Rimmel Cool Blue pencil

EYES, FILL IN FLAME blue from Ben Nye wheel (see page 62)

FOUNDATION Trûcco Porcelain Ivory

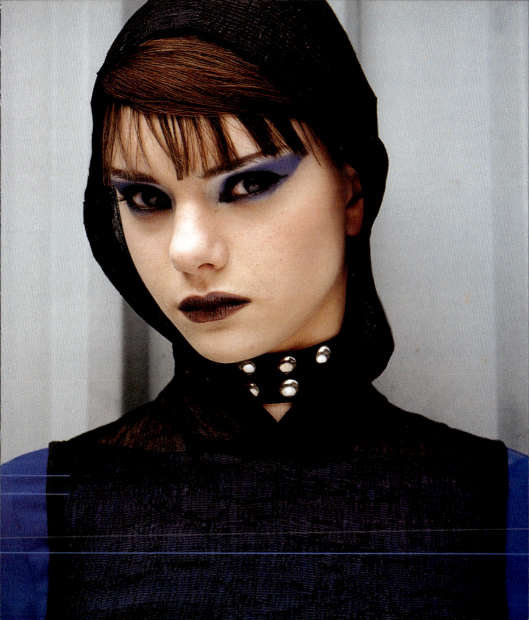

flybrow

THE KIT: rubber stamp with simple design (see page 62), white crayon, gold powder (or Rimmel Liquid Gold eyeliner dabbed onto back of hand), hair grip, red lipstick (or the red from the Ben Nye wheel – see page 62), feathers, eyelash glue (or spirit gum).

Coat the stamp with crayon, dip into your chosen gold, and then press hard onto skin. Repeat until the design is complete. Dip the end of a hair grip into your chosen red to dot the design. Stick feathers gently to eyebrows with the glue.

EYES Trūcco Preem

LIPS Trūcco diVinyls Black Dahlia

CHEEKS Trūcco Flirt

FOUNDATION Trūcco Porcelain Bisque

HIGHLIGHT CHEEK BONES, BROW AND NOSE
Colourings highlighter stick Asteroid

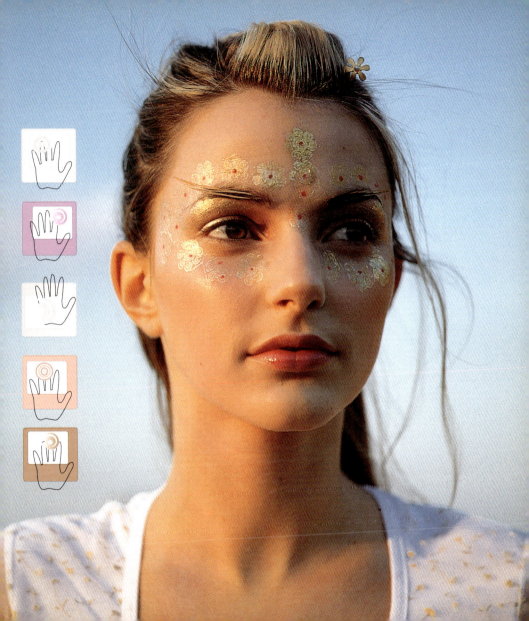

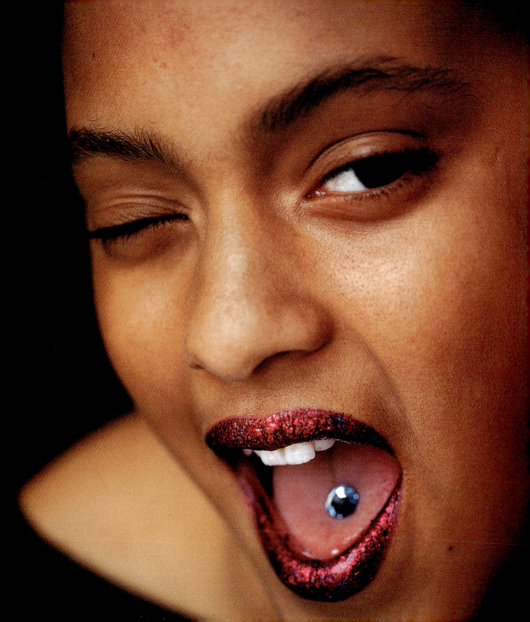

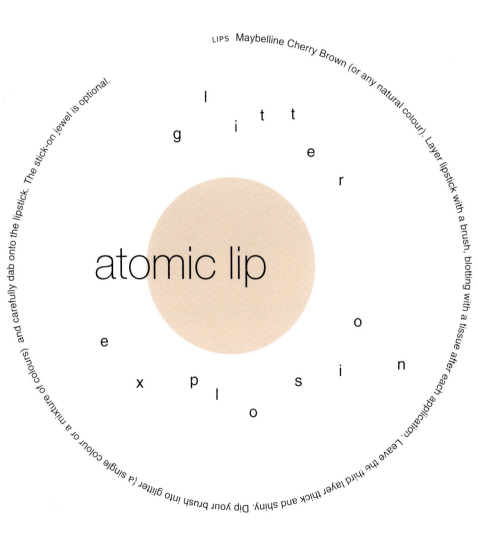

atomic lip

glitter explosion

LIPS Maybelline Cherry Brown (or any natural colour). Layer lipstick with a brush, blotting with a tissue after each application. Leave the third layer thick and shiny. Dip your brush into glitter (a single colour or a mixture of colours) and carefully dab onto the lipstick. The stick-on jewel is optional.

LIGHT FORCE

CHEEKS FOREHEAD AND JAWBONE
Maybelline Great Wear blush Toffee-caramel

EYES Colourings Tex Mex Yellow

EYES Max Factor
EarthSpirits Barleyfields and
Max Factor Earth Spirits Terrafirma

EYES   yellow and orange from
Ben Nye wheel (see page 62)

LIPS Colourings
lipshine pencil, Lilac

NOSE yellow from Ben Nye wheel and
Max Factor Wicked White pencil

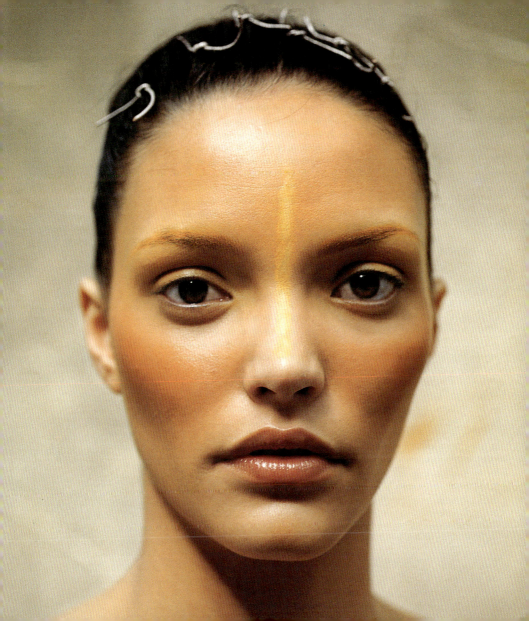

White Wash

FOUNDATION
Max Factor Sheer Genius

CHEEKS
Maybelline Great Wear Toffee Caramel

EYES
Colourings Oyster Pearl

EYES
Colourings Golden Pearl

UNDER EYE
Colourings Oatmeal

HIGHLIGHT CHEEK BONES, BROW AND NOSE
Colourings Oyster Pearl

LIPS
Rimmel Paradise

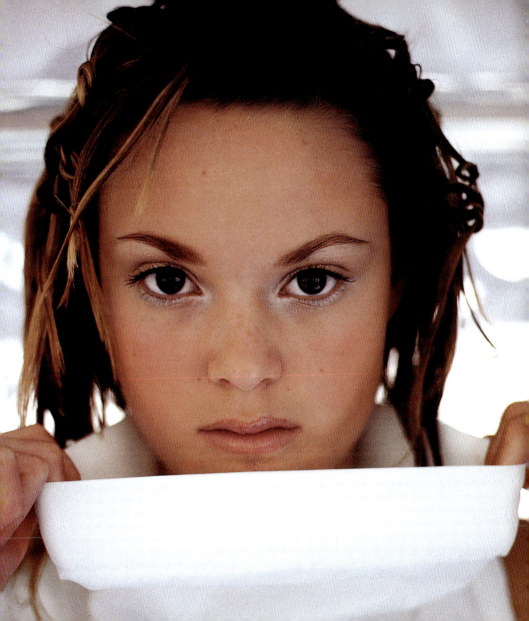

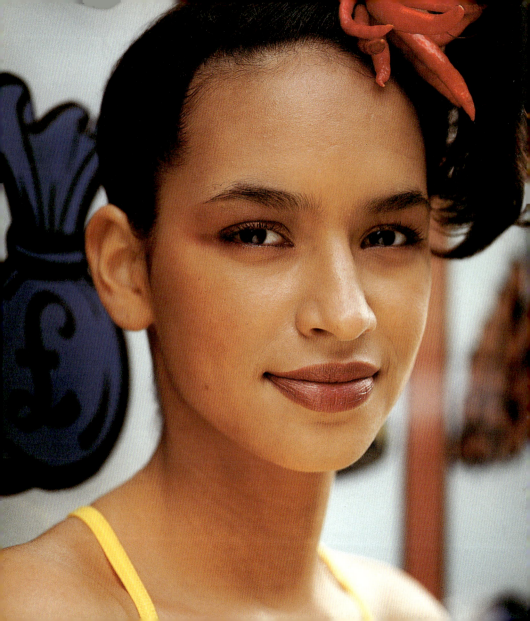

Max Factor Earth Spirits Heat

EYES Trücco Tribal Reflective

EYES Trücco Tribal Reflective

ALL OVER FACE Trücco Jewel compact

ALL OVER FACE Trücco Jewel compact

CHEEKS AND BROW Trücco Jewel compact

LIPS Trücco Fatal

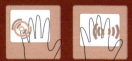
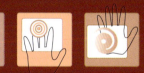

chilli

Vinyl Fusion

FOUNDATION
Max Factor 3-in-1 complete makeup Fair

EYES Vaseline

EYES
Max Factor Earth Spirits Onyx

EYES
Rimmel Jet Black eye pencil

CHEEKS
Maybelline Great Wear blush

LIPS MAC gel

MASCARA Rimmel Endless Lash Black

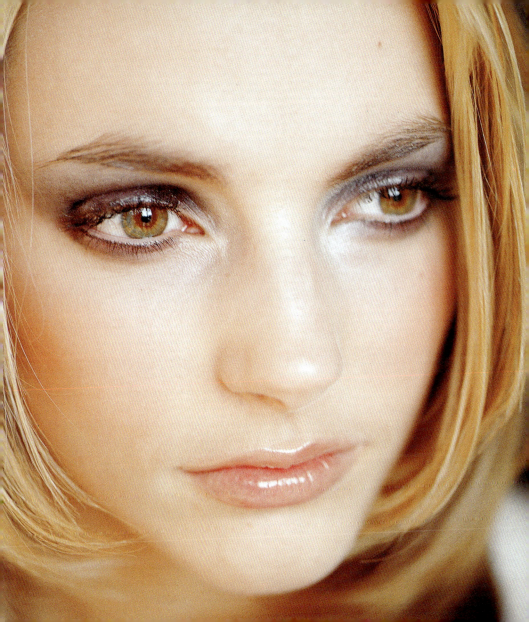

THE KIT: ruler, neutral lip pencil, heart-shaped sequins (see page 62), eyelash glue or spirit gum (see page 62), tweezers.

Using the ruler, draw a line across the cheeks and nose with the lip pencil.

Starting from the nose, and working out towards the edge of the face, stick sequins on top of the line with eyelash glue (or gum).

Use only a little glue at a time, and tweezers for accuracy.

Tribal Heart

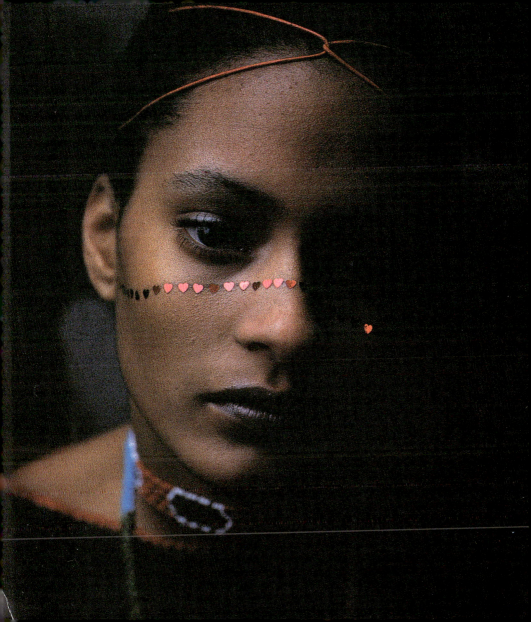

useful items

All products used within this book are available at the time of going to press, although products can be replaced with similar colours and items from any range.

The items listed here will be useful when creating a number of the looks contained in this book, and will hopefully inspire further experimentation and individual design.

BEN NYE RAINBOW WHEEL
This is a small compact containing segments of blue, red, yellow, green, orange and black stage make-up, much like greasepaint. Extremely versatile, this can be used whenever strong, matte colour is required.

BEN NYE CLOWN WHITE
With the texture of greasepaint, this can be used for more theatrical looks, to get a strong, matte white base.

BHINDIS, JEWELS, SEQUINS, AND STICK-ON ACCESSORIES
Originally a mark of religious and cultural significance in Asian communities, bhindis have gradually filtered into the fashion world. Spectacular Cosmetics has a very large range, and speciality store Daminis offers mail-order. Accessories can also be found in many high street stores nationwide.

EYELASH GLUE OR SPIRIT GUM
Eyelash glue can be found (packaged with false eyelashes) in Boots, Superdrug and independent chemists. Shuuemura sell glue as a separate product. Spirit gum can be found in any art supply store.

GLITTER
This comes in myriad colours for both body and face. Although widely available, one of the best stockists, with a full range of colours, is Spectacular Cosmetics.

GOLD LEAF
Available from any art supply store.

L'ORÉAL ID IDENTITÉ MEHNDI KIT
This little package includes a liner brush with black and white inkwells, step-by-step instructions on how to use a stencil to create body decoration, a simple stencil to get you started, and suggestions for patterns and motifs for freehand design.

RUBBER STAMPS
Available from Blade Rubber, these are small blocks of wood with stuck-on rubber designs. They can be used as part of any design on face or body.

STENCILS
Available from Spectacular Cosmetics in a variety of designs, and as part of the L'Oréal Mehndi kit, these can be used again and again for applying a pattern or motif to the skin.

where to buy

BEN NYE
Available from Screenface (24 Powis Terrace, London W11 1JH; 48 Monmouth Street London WC2 9EP. Tel: 0171 836 3955; Fax: 0171 836 3944). Information on Screenface is available on the web: www.screenface.com.

For Ben Nye catalogue and mail order: Ben Nye Co. Inc., 5935 Bowcroft St, Los Angeles, CA90016, USA. Tel: 001 310 839 1984.

BLADE RUBBER
Offers a mail order service and will also create stamps to order from an original design. For information: 2 Neals Yard, LONDON, WC2H 9DP. Tel: 0171 379 7391.

COLOURINGS
Available at all branches of The Body Shop. For information, call customer services: 01903 731500.

You can also visit the Body Shop website, which is interactive with do-it-yourself profiles and a virtual make-over: www.bodyshop.co.uk.

DAMINIS
Available from their stores in London and Leicester, and by mail order. For full details and mail order: 0181 503 4200.

ELIZABETH ARDEN
Available worldwide from leading department stores and independent chemists.

L'ORÉAL
Available worldwide from independent chemists and leading department stores.

MAC
Available from the two London MAC stores (109 King's Road, SW3 4PA; 28 Fouberts Close, W1V 1HG) and department stores worldwide (including Selfridges and Harvey Nichols). Details and mail order: 0171 534 9222.

MAX FACTOR
Available worldwide from high street stores, supermarkets (including Tesco) and chemists.

MAYBELLINE
Available from most chemists, including Superdrug and Boots, and leading department stores worldwide.

RIMMEL
Available at Boots, Superdrug, and Woolworths, and chemists nationwide. For information: 01233 62 5076.

SPECTACULAR COSMETICS
For glitter and accessories in all colours and designs: no single item costs more than £3. For full information: 0181 903 2020; or e-mail: sales@spectacular.co.uk.

TRŪCCO SEBASTIAN
Available worldwide through appointed professional hair salons. For stockists and mail order: 01256 351188 (UK) or 001 818 999 5112 (USA).

acknowledgements

The publishers would like to thank the following stores:
ACCESSORIZE: hairband (Making Waves); **THE BEAD SHOP:** jewellery (Tribal Heart); **BELLA FREUD:** black and pink top (Cosmic Eye Ray); **B GIRLS:** denim tops (Tribal Heart); **BIBA:** denim jacket (Digital Eye Movement), orange top (Free Spirit), bronze top (Vinyl Fusion); **CONCIOUS EARTHWEAR:** white top (White Wash), red fleece (Rad Red), blue jacket (Rush), grey fleece (Metal Ice); **FLYJACK:** silver top and combat trousers (Making Waves), black top (Light Force); **GOLDIE:** blue top (Metal Ice), blue top (Wicked); **THE HAT SHOP:** red hat (Rad Red), green hat (Free Spirit); **HENNES:** hairclips (Heatwave), choker (Wicked); **KLEINS:** jewel on tongue (Atomic Lip), hairbands (Tribal Heart), hair beading (Freckles), string in hair (Light Force); **MISS SIXTY:** yellow jacket and top (Summer Breeze), navy top (Rush), blue dress (Heatwave), purple top (Atomic Lip), scarf on head (Freckles), yellow vest (Chilli); **MORGAN:** pink top (Urban Angel), white top (Mesmerise), white top (Flybrow); **RED OR DEAD:** black top (Wicked); **SUPERDRUG:** rain hat (Digital Eye Movement); **SUSAN DILLON AT HYPE DF:** lilac dress (Kaleidoscope); **TOP SHOP:** hair clip (Flybrow).

Our thanks also to the models and model agencies involved:
ELITE PREMIER New Faces;
GOODFELLA'S; MODELS 1 New Faces;
STORM New Faces

Thank you to Alice Bonni, Jo Harris, Katharine Lazenby, and Morgana Robinson, for their useful comments and genuine enthusiasm.

author's acknowledgements

To Anne McKevitt, who had true faith in me from the beginning, I offer my grateful thanks; she inspired me to be focussed and to believe in myself. My thanks also to Sam Remer for putting together the perfect clothing and accessories.

Publishing Director: Anne Furniss
Art Director: Helen Lewis
Project Editor: Nicki Marshall
Design: Coralie Bickford-Smith
Production: Julie Hadingham

First published in 1999 by
Quadrille Publishing Limited,
Alhambra House,
27-31 Charing Cross Road,
London WC2H 0LS

Text © 1999 Dennie Pasion
Photographs © 1999 Ursula Steiger
Design & Layout © 1999 Quadrille Publishing Ltd

The rights of Dennie Pasion to be identified as Author of this Work have been asserted by her in accordance with the Copyright, Designs and Patents Act 1988.

All rights reserved. No part of this book may be reproduced, stored in a retrieval system or transmitted in any form or by any means, electronic, electrostatic, magnetic, tape, mechanical, photocopying, recording or otherwise, without the prior permission of the publisher.

Cataloguing in Publication Data:
a catalogue record for this book is available from the British library.

ISBN 1 899988 94 7

Printed in Hong Kong